GREAT

SEX

76 ways to please, tease, excite and ignite

SOURCEBOOKS CASABLANCA™
AN IMPRINT OF SOURCEBOOKS, INC.®
NAPERVILLE, ILLINOIS

NOTES

JOHN LESLIE WOLFE

Published by Sourcebooks, Inc.
P.O. Box 4410, Naperville, Illinois 60567-4410
(630) 961-3900
FAX: (630) 961-2168
www.sourcebooks.com

   Library of Congress Cataloging-in-Publication Data

Wolfe, John Leslie.
  Great sex notes : 76 ways to please, tease, excite and ignite / John Leslie Wolfe.
      p. cm.
  Includes bibliographical references.
  ISBN 1-4022-0545-7 (alk. paper)
  1. Sex instruction for women. 2. Sex instruction for men. I. Title: Great Sex Notes. II. Title.

HQ46.W63 2005
613.9'6—dc22

                                        2005017688

             Printed and bound in the United States of America
                    SP 10 9 8 7 6 5 4 3 2 1

INTRODUCTION

There are countless books on how to be a great lover, on great seduction, on how to and why to. Many of those books say that communication is the key to good sex. However, communication is where most of us need help. Most of us know the mechanics of sex and basically what we enjoy. Letting our partner know what we want, how we are feeling that day, is often complicated by worry about how our partner will feel, timing, and differing moods.

The purpose of this book is to facilitate communication. It is filled with very simple notes for you to leave your partner, with suggestions of what is on your mind or what you think might be fun for the two of you to try. It is meant to simplify sometimes-difficult conversations about sex, and to introduce some variety into the routine that most couples fall into. No props are needed, no elaborate planning is required. All that is needed is for you to match a note with your mood, and let that note be the starting point for an evening, afternoon, or morning of mutual pleasure.

The premise is that if one partner knows what the other partner wants, or is thinking about, it is good for both.

There are several ways that you can use this book. You can alternate turns presenting a note. You can each present a note at the same time. You can present multiple notes. You can leave them to be found later, hand them to one another personally, or thumb through the book together to look for inspiration. It really doesn't matter. These notes are just to get you started. How you finish, or if you finish, is entirely up to you.

However, if your partner suggests, with his or her note, something that you really feel you don't want to do, just say so, with as little opinion as possible. Maybe say, "Let's save that one, and pick another one for now." Mostly, just play and have fun learning more about your friend and lover.

USING YOUR GREAT SEX NOTES

The first half of each page is a basic explanation, or information about the note alongside it, that would seem useful to one or both of you. All of the pages are identified as to which partner it applies to, but if you can find other ways to use them, great. *Great Sex Notes* is meant to help you communicate and to inspire some fun, some playfulness, and some great sex.

The notes are separated, with her notes in the first half, and his in the second half. Use them all or just a few. Repeat the ones you like the best. Whatever is your pleasure.

Keep in mind that a note left ahead of time will provide hours of pleasant anticipation for both of you.

Enjoy!

HAND MASSAGE

Hands are remarkable, and so often they are overworked and neglected. One of the most relaxing and sensual things you can do for your lover is to massage his hands. Don't worry about technique. It's hard to go wrong. Near the end of the day, when it's quiet and the distractions have ended, or just as you go to bed, take whatever lotion you have on hand, and just massage his hands. Stretch them, bend them, and gently pull his fingers. Rub between his fingers and onto his forearm, almost to his elbow. Three or four minutes on each hand will feel amazing to him.

You can move on to lovemaking or not. But your generosity won't be forgotten.

This evening, I want to give you a hand massage...

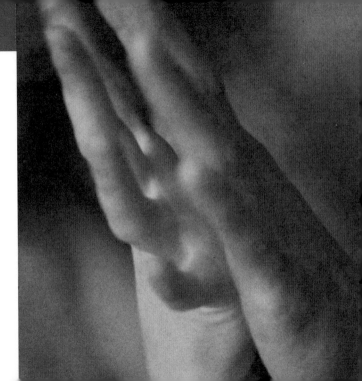

HAND MASSAGE

When the day has ended, when it's quiet, I will relax you with some attention to your hard working hands. Just lie back, close your eyes, and enjoy the relaxation. Afterward, you can doze off, if you like, or you can let those relaxed hands roam around my body. Your choice.

BALL ONE, BALL TWO

Here is a gift your man won't soon forget. Your next love-making session will be dedicated to his "fellas," his "boys," his testicles.

You might be reluctant to handle them much, having heard all the jokes over the years about how fragile they are. Like women's breasts, they are sometimes tender, but overall, they are quite sturdy and rather neglected.

Handle them, lift them up, grasp his whole scrotum, and pull them easily downward. Suck one gently into your mouth. He has fantasized about that, I promise you. He'll let you know if you get too rough, but the idea of your handling this most intimate part of his anatomy will be an amazing turn on.

Tonight, I want to give my full attention to your balls...

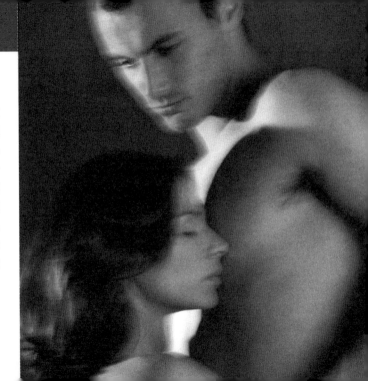

BALL ONE, BALL TWO

Tonight, my darling, I want to give my full attention to your testicles, your balls, your "boys." Coach me, if I need any help, and tell me if I play too rough. But I want you to just lie back and enjoy the attention.

THE BREAST JOB

Men love breasts. Period. They are simply wonderful, no matter what their shape or size.

So, what better idea than during your next lovemaking session, you give your man your full attention with only your breasts. Once you have gotten started, ask him to lie back with his hands at his sides, while you rub your breasts over his entire body. Work your way down his chest, his legs and arms, and his back. Then rub his penis with your breasts. Move up his chest and rub his face, just with your breasts. Rub his eyes and lips with your nipples. He won't be able to get enough of that. At about that point, he will probably have trouble keeping his hands at his side any longer. His mouth and hands will want to join in the fun.

I know you like my breasts…

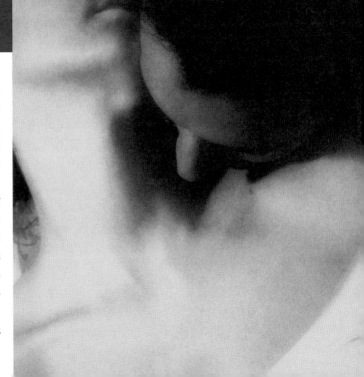

THE BREAST JOB

I know you like my breasts, so I am going to use them to stroke your entire body. I am going to rub them up and down your chest and back, your arms and legs. Then I will stroke your penis with my breasts, touch your nipples with mine, and rub my breasts on your face. With my nipples, I will stroke your eyelids and lips.

That should get us started nicely.

BATH TIME

Tonight invite your man to join you for a relaxing bath. Light a candle and pour a glass of wine, if you wish, to slow down the moment and add to the ceremony. Run plenty of warm water, get out the bubble bath, and ask him to meet you. Then take a cloth and wash him. Have him sit in front of you and wash his back. Invite him to stand, and wash his legs, ass, and finally, his penis. If you want, have him sit behind you, hand him the cloth, and let him follow your example. Or, you can save that. A future sex note puts you on the receiving end of the wash cloth. In the meantime, this night will be off to a good *clean* start.

Join me in my warm, wet bath…

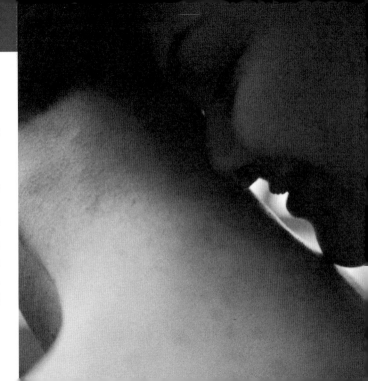

BATH TIME

This evening, I would love it if you would join me for a relaxing, yet stimulating bath. When we're ready to wind down from the day, I'll get the water ready, and you can pour us a glass of wine, if you like. Then you can join me in the nice warm water. Sit in front of me, I'll wash your back...and more.

LOCATION, LOCATION

Now, if you are the adventuresome type, you may be way ahead of this one, but every couple falls into routines. The bedroom is a wonderful place for lovemaking, but wouldn't a change of scenery be interesting? Let him pick the place, or you decide, but find someplace where you've never made love before. That way, every time either of you passes that place, you will think of the intimate moment you had there. Whether you pick a hallway, the laundry room, or the kitchen table, that place will hold a special memory, and you will have had an adventure.

Let's make love someplace new....

LOCATION, LOCATION

The next time we make love, my darling, I want it to be someplace we have never made love before. I love our bed, but let's try a new place—on the floor of the hallway, on the kitchen table, in the closet—it doesn't matter. Just pick a place and lead me there. I have a couple of ideas, if you need inspiration.

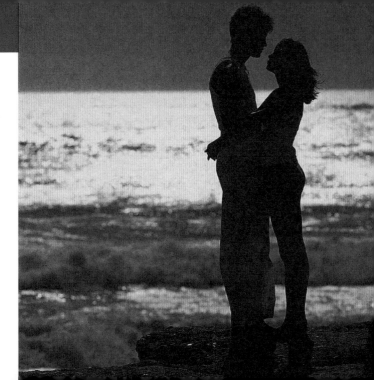

COME AS YOU WISH

Orgasms have a life of their own, but we fall into patterns there, also. For a man, his orgasm can be a very exciting visual stimulant, in addition to the great physical pleasure of the moment itself. So, the next time you make love, give him the permission to come wherever he wants. Of course, you know what your birth control and safety needs are, and the two of you will maintain those. But, fearing that you could have a negative opinion, he might be reluctant to tell you that he would love to come on your breasts, or your stomach, or your feet, or on some other favorite body part. He'll be very excited knowing you're inviting him to try a fantasy.

Wherever you want to come...

COME AS YOU WISH

Darling, as we near the end of our lovemaking tonight, I invite you to come wherever you wish. You can stay inside me, or you can come on my breasts, my stomach, or your favorite spot on my body. Spend the day thinking about that, and tonight "come as you wish." We'll have a nice warm towel to dry off with afterward and then we can drift off to sleep.

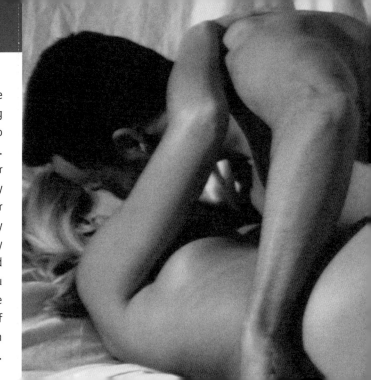

BJ

This one can be good for both of you. Give him this note, but then surprise—don't wait for the usual bedtime. He'll know it's coming, but when? When the moment seems right, stop him where he is, or, even better, take him by the hand and lead him to a place with a mirror. Kiss him, then slowly kneel and begin. Men have preferences for what feels best at a given moment, so encourage him to guide you, in terms of harder or softer. Your hand wrapped around his penis, between your mouth and his body, can greatly increase his pleasure, help you control how deep in your mouth you wish him to be, and allow you to jack him off and suck him at the same time. It will be a thrilling experience for him.

I want you in my mouth...

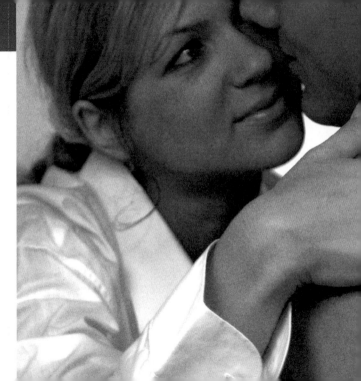

BJ

I want you. I want you in my mouth. How do the words, "Would you like a blow job?" sound? That's what I want you to have. I know you'll like what I do, but to be sure, I want you to guide me and tell me if you want me to be faster or slower, to suck you harder or softer.

You...in my mouth ...tonight...

EXPLORE ME

Remember the very early days of your being a couple, and the excitement of the exploration and discovery. There was something in the buildup and anticipation that exists before you become accustomed to one another's bodies. Tonight, relive those early times.

Instead of your usual routines of getting ready for bed, invite him to undress you. Recreate the excitement of those early days. Turn the lights low and set a mood, then let him take everything off of you. When you are naked, allow him to use his eyes and fingertips to go over every inch of you. To explore the places not usually concentrated on. To notice your curves. To trace the small of your back. He'll love being able to celebrate your body, and you'll love the memory of being explored for the first time, again.

Explore every inch of me…

EXPLORE ME

Tonight let's go back in time to when anticipation was so much of the excitement. I want you to slowly undress me, take everything off me.

I want you to explore me with your fingers and eyes. Notice the small of my back, my hair, the curve under my breast. Trace the backs of my knees, and explore my nipples. Then, take off your clothes and enjoy your new discovery.

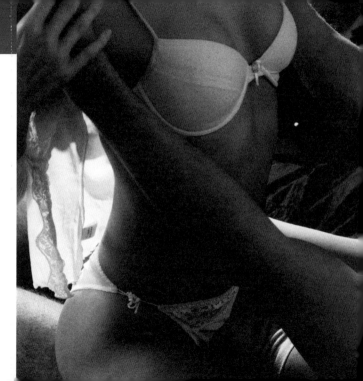

WATCH ME

It's no secret that men are highly visual. You may or may not be completely comfortable being naked in front of him, but he loves seeing you. You can combine the pleasure of seeing you naked and the total erotic excitement he will have of watching you touch yourself with an educational experience. By letting him watch you touch yourself, you will be helping him to learn how you like to be touched, and giving him a highly exciting experience at the same time, an experience he has fantasized about many times.

Once you are in bed together, invite him to sit back and enjoy the view. Use your hands to explore your own body as you like. Don't think of it as a performance, but as a moment of self-pleasure. You can make it last as long as you like. He will be breathless and happy. When, finally, you ask him to join you, he will be more than ready.

Just watch....

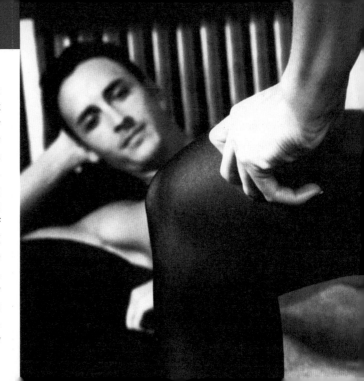

WATCH ME

Tonight, my love, I'm going to lie back and let my hands roam over my body. I want you to enjoy watching my hands as they caress my breasts, and then enjoy watching as my fingers move down to find the soft places of pleasure. Watch how I move my hands, and the pleasure it brings me. After awhile, I'll surely want your hands to join mine, but until then, just lie back and enjoy the view.

TOUCH ME AS I DO

Tonight, you are going to combine the elements of self-pleasure and massage, allowing your man to give you the attention you enjoy. After you are in bed, let him sit back behind you. Sit in front of him, lean back and let his hands reach around and become your hands. Let his hands roam over your body and caress you in the ways that you enjoy. He wants to know how to please you, so gently coach him as to where his hands should go next, where and how fast you want his fingers to move. Relax, and let him focus entirely on your pleasure. It will be his pleasure, as well.

Let your hands become my hands…

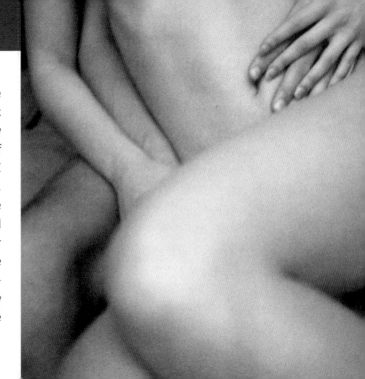

TOUCH ME AS I DO

The next time we are together in bed, I want your hands to become my hands. Make yourself comfortable on the bed. I will sit in front of you. Put your arms around me and caress me as I would myself. Pretend your hands are mine. We'll take our time, and together— with your hands and my body—we'll touch all the right places.

A SPECIAL MASSAGE

You always touch each other when you make love, but this time, make it a point to pay slow and deliberate attention to his penis, in the form of a massage. This isn't a hand job. You are not even going to bring him to orgasm. It is just focused attention on that part of him. Make a point to have some oil near by, and after you are comfortable together, wet your hands with the oil and take hold of him. Rub the oil into the area around his penis, massage his balls gently, and then grip the shaft of his penis and slowly move your hands up and down. Again, the intent is not to bring him to orgasm, but just to let you both focus on the sensations of your massage. The pleasure you bring him will intensify everything that follows.

A small but very special massage...

A SPECIAL MASSAGE

When we make love tonight, I am going to stop briefly and ask you to lie back. I am going to take your penis in my hands and give you a slow, gentle massage. Enjoy the sensation. It's not about you coming, just focused energy on that area of your body. We can move on from there, if we like, but for those few moments, just lie there...feel my hands ...moving gently.

CONTROL #1

You spend the day managing your time and your business and your life and your home. Sometimes, you just don't want to manage anything else. Tonight, let him take complete control in the bedroom. Let him set the lights, the mood, the clothing, the music, and let him guide you physically. Be passive, and see where he takes you.

You take control tonight...

CONTROL #1

Sometimes, my darling, I get tired of planning or even thinking. I think I'll take a little mental vacation. But I still want to make love. So tonight, at bedtime, I want you to plan the lights, location, what I wear, and where you want me. I intend to take part in every way I just don't want to be in charge of anything except taking pleasure from you.

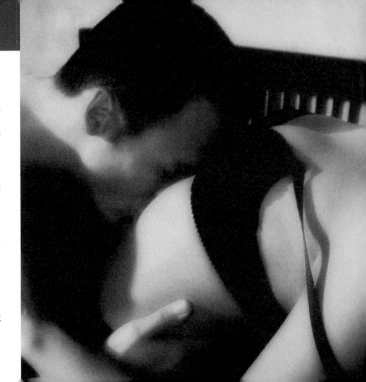

CONTROL #2

Of course, there are times when giving over control, even to your dearest one, is the last thing on your mind. There are days when your mental and physical desires combine powerfully, but you might be unsure about letting him know that. On the other hand, men often feel that they are expected to be assertive. Knowing that tonight you want to take that role for yourself will be a treat for him and an adventure for you.

I'll take control tonight....

CONTROL #2

I know that your day is sometimes stressful, and by the time we get to bed you just want to escape. Tonight, just show up. You won't have to think about anything. Be as passive as you want, without feeling any need to please me, or to lead our activities in bed. You don't have to do anything other than follow my lead and enjoy our mutual pleasure.

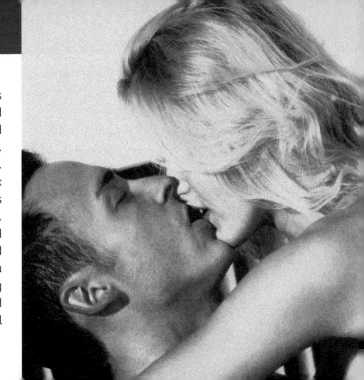

ANY ROOM IN THE SHOWER?

For a man, a shower is mostly just for getting clean. But most men recognize the sensuous possibilities of their shower, and have often wished you were in there with them. In fact, if you want to see your man smile, just step into his shower and ask, "May I join you?"

So, tonight, take advantage of a frequent fantasy of his, and start—or finish—the evening with some wet, warm, and soapy attention to your body. Be prepared to get your hair wet, and have a nice time.

I'll keep you company in the shower…

ANY ROOM IN THE SHOWER?

Darling, I think I'll join you when you shower— there are a few spots I'm having a hard time reaching by myself. Take your bare hands, and some soap, and slowly wash my back. Slowly wash all the way down my backside, to my legs, and then turn me around and wash my breasts and my stomach and...so on. That should give us a nice clean start to the rest of the evening.

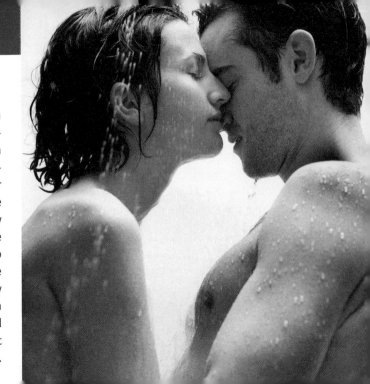

TOUCH ME OTHER PLACES

Couples that have been together for any length of time can fall into patterns of lovemaking. That is, they caress one another in similar ways each time they make love. At the risk of generalizing, men are probably quicker to fall into a pattern of going for the hot spots right away, forgetting about some of the subtler areas that might have been explored earlier in your relationship.

With this sex note, suggest to your partner that he completely avoid touching you between your legs or on your nipples, at least until you ask him to. Instead, he should use his hands anywhere and everywhere else. You know that you have plenty of erotic zones on your body, and they surely need more attention.

I love the feeling of your fingers…

TOUCH ME OTHER PLACES

Darling, I love when you touch me, exploring my nipples and between my legs. But tonight, I want you to avoid touching either of those places. Instead, explore the many other places on my body that love your touch—my legs, stomach, cheeks of my ass, neck, and insides of my thighs. Let your fingers explore my skin. Don't let your fingers actually touch my nipples or caress between my legs...until I urge you to.

KISS ME OTHER PLACES

In the same way that you and your partner's hands tend to travel familiar territory, your kisses also seem to find the same places over and over again. As lovely as that is, with this sex note encourage him to do with his lips as you have encouraged him to do with his hands. That is, as you make love, he should explore your body with his kisses, but should avoid the most obvious and familiar places. Again, at least until you urge him to.

Kiss every part of my body…

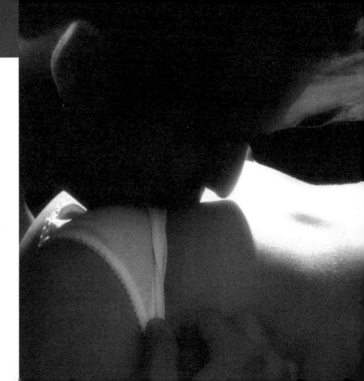

KISS ME OTHER PLACES

I love your kisses on my body. Tonight I offer you a challenge. I want you to find places that your lips have not gotten to know well. Nibble and kiss your way around the back of my neck and knees, the soles of my feet, my eyelids, the insides of my thighs, between my fingers, and down my back. Explore me with your lips. I can't wait.

I'LL WATCH YOU

Most men are fairly comfortable with touching themselves erotically. The idea of masturbating, not only with your permission, but also with your involvement, will be extremely exciting for him. For you, it will allow you to share sex with your man on an evening when you might not feel like full intercourse, and it will allow you to learn more about how your man likes to be aroused. We can each learn from seeing how our partner treats their own body. He will love the idea that on a night when you might not really feel like sex, you still want him to have pleasure. Of course, you might decide that you want to get involved, once you see things getting under way.

I want to watch you....

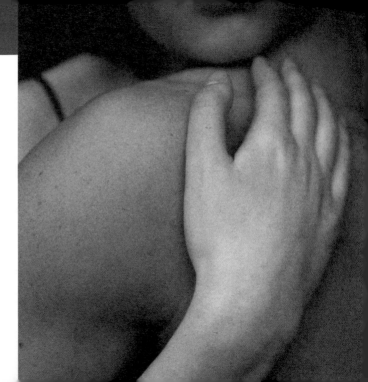

I'LL WATCH YOU

Honey, I want to watch you. If you want help getting underway, I'll be more than happy to provide assistance. But then, I want to sit back and witness your pleasure. I want to see how you grip yourself, and see how you move your hands faster or slower. I want to learn from you and see the pleasure you feel as you come.

WITHOUT A TOP

These facts are fairly undisputed: men are visual, and they enjoy seeing breasts. Innumerable products are sold employing just that premise. And how many strip clubs and men's magazines exist just to capitalize on those facts? But the breasts he likes most are yours. He thinks about them many times a day, and if you would show them to him right now, he would be a happy man.

Although it may not seem erotic or exciting to you, your man has often thought about how nice it would be if you were topless during otherwise non-sexual moments. He has fantasized about having you be topless during dinner, or while you watch TV together, or at some other moment that might surprise you.

Tonight, offer him the pleasure of enjoying this fantasy.

Topless time...

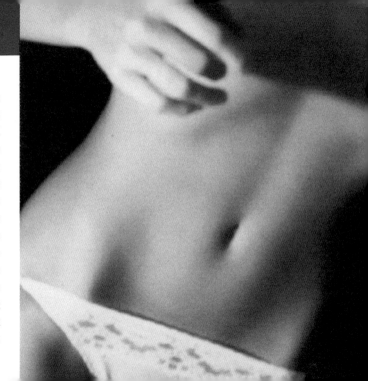

WITHOUT A TOP

You know I have gotten the impression that you enjoy my breasts. So, I think I'll spend a little nonsexual time with you...topless. You'll have to let me know when you might think it would be enjoyable. Our options would include dinnertime, or maybe while we watch TV. Just a little treat for your eyes, but you can let me know if it brings any other activities to mind.

MAKE OUT

Some of these notes are to help you move forward, some of them are to help you move backward. If you have been a couple for awhile, some of the early courtship rituals have been left behind, along with the anticipation and excitement that accompanied them. When was the last time the two of you made out, nowhere near a bed, and without knowing it would lead to sex?

With this note, suggest to your partner that you find a place other than bed, and make out. Whether you move on to sex or not, is entirely up to the two of you. But try to recall a time when making out was the end in itself.

Let's make out....

MAKE OUT

Remember the early days in our relationship when our kisses were so sexually charged, before we knew each other's bodies? Let's recreate that tonight. We'll meet on the sofa, on the back porch, or in the back seat of the car. We'll kiss for kissing's sake. Of course, it might lead us to bed, but first, let's just find a nice spot and make out.

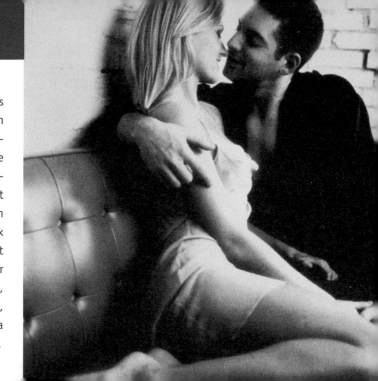

NO HANDS, PLEASE

This will be a challenge for you both, although a pleasurable and imaginative one. The next time you make love, invite him to join you in using every part of your bodies, except for your hands. Not only will it change any routines you have in your lovemaking, it will also bring awareness to the possibilities found in other parts of your bodies, and almost certainly provide some fun and exercise your imaginations.

Look, lover, no hands....

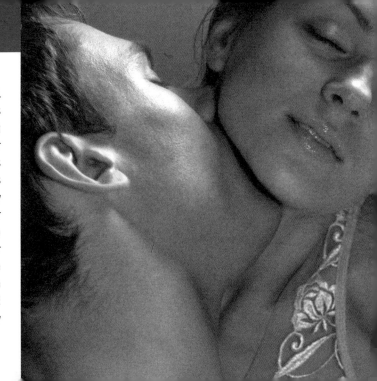

NO HANDS, PLEASE

I offer you this sexual challenge, my dear. Let's have a wonderful evening of sex without using our hands. The possibilities are endless. I can caress you with my hair and my breasts, or massage your ass with mine. You can tickle my back with your nose, rub my ass with your feet, my nipples with your penis. Our lips and tongues will be very busy. But, no hands.

WHO'S WATCHING WHOM?

There are times, when you are making love, that you would like to slow down a bit, just to catch your breath. Or, you would like to extend the moment and not get to the finale too soon. In either case, the goal is to intensify an already exciting evening.

You can slow down and intensify the experience at the same time. The next time you are making love, as you feel the intensity building, take a break. Sit back from one another and for your own pleasure, and the visual pleasure of your partner, slowly please your own bodies. Do those things that please you when you are alone. Sharing what is usually an exciting, but solitary experience will thrill him. After a few moments, move back together, and resume your lovemaking, with renewed excitement.

Who's watching?...

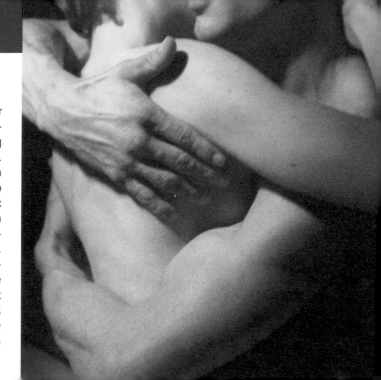

WHO'S WATCHING WHOM?

My dear one, no matter how long it lasts, sometimes our lovemaking doesn't seem long enough. The next time, when things are feeling so nice, I'm going to ask you to pause. We'll each sit back and take pleasure in our own bodies. We'll touch only ourselves and watch, as we slow our lovemaking, yet build our excitement. A brief and very enjoyable rest, before our bodies resume their rhythm.

A TRIBUTE TO VICTORIA'S SECRET

Men love lingerie. He may not mention it, but he does notice and takes great interest in your intimate apparel.

I have tried to keep these sex notes simple and cost-free. But this one exception should bring each of you pleasure.

For a man, the idea of buying lingerie is filled with confusion and complexity. He wonders if you will like what he gets for you, and more than anything else, dealing with the sizes stops him in his tracks.

Help him. Give him your exact sizes. He may not select the same thing that you would, and it's unlikely he'll buy you something sensible. This is just for fun—and who knows, he might get you something quite nice.

The next time you find yourself walking by a lingerie department, I want you to know my sizes…just in case you feel tempted….

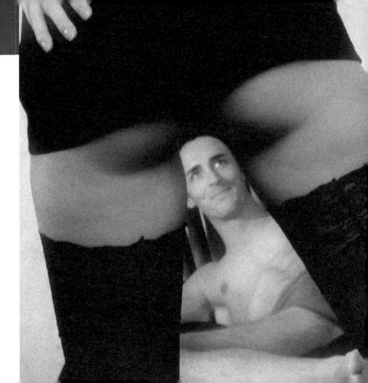

A TRIBUTE TO VICTORIA'S SECRET

Here is all you need:

Bra _____

Panties _____

Garter Belt _____

Stockings _____

Panty Hose _____

Teddy _____

Negligee _____

Underwire? _____
(yes or no)

Thong? _____
(yes or no)

YOUR HANDS, MY BOOTIE

Most men have a favorite part when it comes to women, but your rear end is always a pleasure for him to see and touch. It probably has to do with anthropology, and when we walked on all fours. And whatever you think of your own backside, he gets great pleasure from it.

In fact, your gluteus maximus is more than just something to fill out those new pants you bought or a cushion to sit on. It is also three very large muscles on each side that function to extend, rotate, and otherwise control the thigh.

Now, don't these hard working muscles deserve some attention? He'll love it, and you can let it lead you wherever you want it to.

My dear, my backside gets nice attention from you, but it might need a little more. I would love having you massage my bottom.

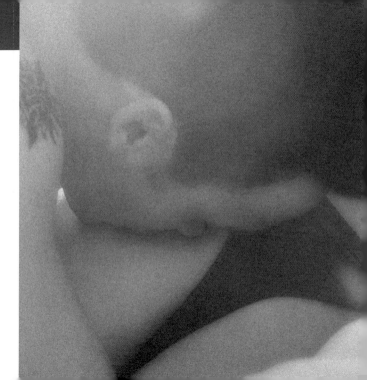

YOUR HANDS, MY BOOTIE

Your hands on my back-side will feel so good. Use oil and work the muscles of my ass with long, slow strokes. Run your thumbs up and down between my buns and gently circle the opening. Let your index finger circle and massage my opening, but just let the tip of your finger enter slightly. Let the palm of your other hand reach under me and press against my pubic hair, moving in a circle. Hmmm...nice.

NOT YET...WAIT FOR IT

If you are like most people these days, you are always rushed and often tired. Added to our being creatures of habit, that often means that in our sex lives we move to the main event almost immediately. What is left of foreplay, for many established couples, is just the bare minimum of what it takes to get the engines running.

This whole book is meant to get people to communicate more and break their sexual routines. This sex note will return you to earlier, more imaginative days.

You will need a timing device—an alarm, kitchen timer, something. Together, decide on a length of time: 10, 15, or 20 minutes. Once you begin making love, agree that there will be no intercourse until that time has passed. For most couples, 10 or 15 minutes of foreplay will be quite an enjoyable change.

It may not be easy, but wait for it.

Take your time...

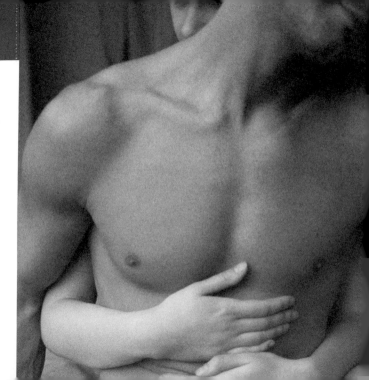

NOT YET...WAIT FOR IT

Darling, we are busy, we are rushed, and as much as I love the sex we have together, we have both slipped in the foreplay department.

So, here's what we'll do. I have a timer. Tonight, we'll select 10, 15, or 20 minutes, and we will not have any penetration until the timer runs out. When that bell goes off...we will too.

UNDRESS ME

When you first became sexual with your partner, perhaps he fumbled hurriedly or maybe proceeded very carefully in getting you out of your clothes. Now that you've been together for awhile, you usually just undress yourselves and meet in bed. What would it be like to bring back some of that anticipation into this wonderful event? What better way than to encourage your partner to completely undress you.

Don't help him, don't suggest when or how, don't finish what you are doing, or go through all of your regular routines beforehand. You can wash your face and rinse out your coffee cup later. I'm not sure which will be more enjoyable, him spending the day knowing that you want him to undress you, or you spending the day knowing that is what he is going to do.

Take off all my clothes...

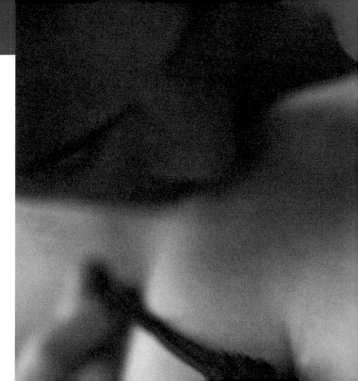

UNDRESS ME

My darling, one of the ceremonies that we neglect these days is that bit of anticipation when the clothes are coming off.

I want you to do something we haven't done in awhile. I want you to undress me completely, before we make love. We'll get your clothes off next and head for the bath, the bed, the floor, or wherever.

Undress me...tonight.

HAND JOB

For so many couples, sex means intercourse, and often, intercourse with little variation. That's a habit that should be broken. Once you are in bed together, invite him to lay back, not think about you or anything else, and just give himself over to the experience. If you don't know what he would prefer (it changes), encourage him to tell you if he wants your hands dry or wet. Old-fashioned water-based creams like Albolene liquefy with the body's warmth and make for a very wet and slippery lubrication. Some men might prefer nothing but your hands.

Squeeze, vary the grip, and let the rhythm build. Alternate slow and fast speeds, and don't forget his testicles. If you press his perineum or insert a very wet finger into his ass to massage his prostate as he nears his climax, he will have an unforgettable orgasm.

My dear, tonight it's just you...and my hands.

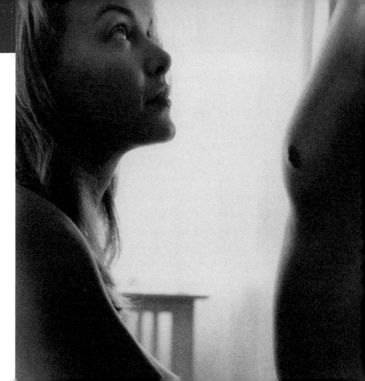

HAND JOB

Seeing you enjoy yourself is the pleasure I need tonight.

You can tell me what you are in the mood for, in terms of whether my hands should be dry or well lubricated. You can help me if you want, either with coaching or with your own hands. But I just want you to lie there, relax, and enjoy the pleasure building until you come.

AURAL SEX

We all hear about how sexy it can be to talk dirty to our partner at the right moment, but being comfortable with it may be another matter. Moods change, but not all men want their lady talking like a sailor, and most men don't really want you to puff them up with a lot of talk about what big studs they are. However, some honest vocal appreciation of him and the sex you share together can be very nice.

Tonight, let him know how he makes you feel, what you want him to do to make you feel good, what you enjoy about his body. You don't have to write a script, or be false. The things he does to you feel good, so just let him know, make some noise, and forget about being a lady. Sex feels just as good to you as it does to anyone. Tonight, you're going to let him know.

Let me tell you how it feels…

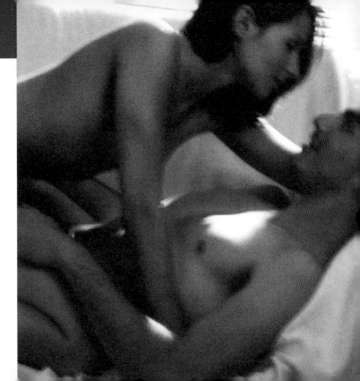

AURAL SEX

When we are in bed together, I don't always express how good you make me feel. Well, the next time, I'm going to let you know.

Tonight, you can expect to hear from me. It may end up with me moaning mostly, but you are going to know that I feel good. I may say, "That feels so good when you.." Or maybe, "I want your.." Or maybe, at the right moment, something really primal and graphic.

ORAL SEX

With the mouths only, that is.

This may seem a challenge, but it's just a little variety for the fun of it. The next time you make love, touch each other with only your mouths. Keep your hands away. Kiss, lick, nibble, and suck all over each other. Try not to use your hands except for support or until you just can't stand not to use them.

It should be a delicious evening.

My mouth...your mouth...your mouth...

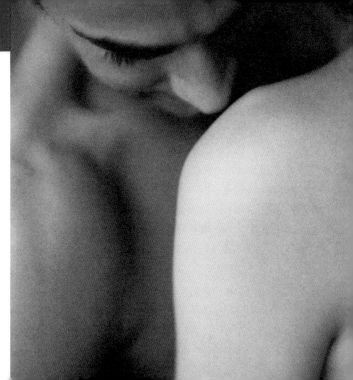

ORAL SEX

Here's a fun challenge for you, my sweet one. I want us to make love with our mouths only. Don't use your hands, and I won't use mine. We'll let our mouths roam where our hands would otherwise. Brush your lips along my neck, run your tongue down my spine, nibble the curve under my breasts, and draw circles on my stomach with your tongue. And, of course...

Let's see, what can I think of for you?

SATURDAY FOR SURE

For some couples, there is a question of when to make love. If one of you is not in the mood that night, it can add pressure or doubt to a relationship. An excellent solution is to pick one night a week that is date night no matter what.

As an experiment, agree on one day of the week, barring illness or emergencies, that the two of you will meet for sex. Don't let anything interfere, not even a bad mood, because each of you has to be able to depend on that meeting. If one partner really doesn't feel like full sex, then the deal is that you will still help the other to enjoy some sexual pleasure. I hope there are plenty of options in this book to inspire you in that regard.

Our sexy date....

SATURDAY FOR SURE

Sweetheart, I want to propose an experiment to try for one month. I love the sex we have. But like everybody, our schedules are often crazy and it's too easy to put off our lovemaking until later.

So, let's choose one day as our "date night." Unless there is sickness or a real emergency, we will not let that day pass without having sex together. Whatever happens the rest of the week, for one month, we'll absolutely meet on

_____.

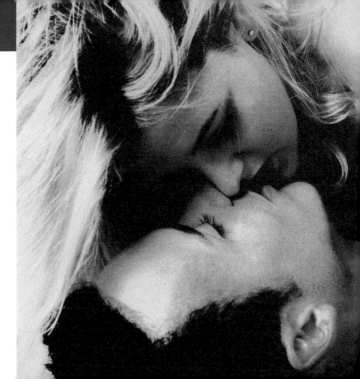

OH, THOSE NAILS

Most people love having their back scratched. So, how about taking that a step further, to a very stimulating variation on a massage. Put those nails to good use.

The next time you make love, give him the treat of slowly and gently scratching his entire body as you begin making love. It will give him the chills. Have him lie on his stomach, and start with his back, making slow circles and long strokes. Lightly scratch his neck and scalp and move down to his ass, legs, and the soles of his feet. Turn him over and repeat the process. Keep the scratching slow and light, but deliberate. Get as close as possible, but wait until last to lightly scratch his penis and balls. Not to tease him, but to build the anticipation.

After scratching him, just smooth his skin with your palms, and proceed naturally.

Let me scratch you...

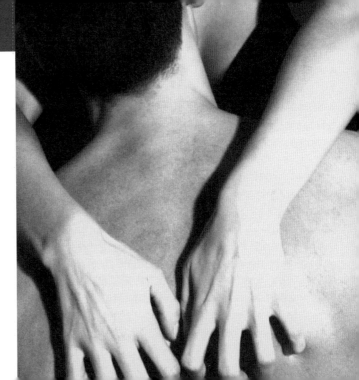

OH, THOSE NAILS

When we are in bed tonight, roll over onto your stomach and I will slowly, and as deliciously as possible, scratch your back, your scalp, your legs, your ass. Then you can roll over so I can lightly scratch your face, your chest, the insides of your thighs...hmmm ...what else?

You might be in dreamland when I finish, or then again, you might be very much awake.

WATER + 6 + 9

Enjoy a bath or shower together. Wash each other, dry each other off, move to the bed and kiss and kiss and all those good things. Then, lying side by side, move into a position for mutual oral sex. Keep it slow. Take your time. Don't seek orgasms, just pleasure. Roll over on top of him so that you can stay in control, and keep the tempo steady but calm. If your own orgasm comes, just relax into it. He'll love it. How you finish the evening is up to you.

Mutual pleasure....

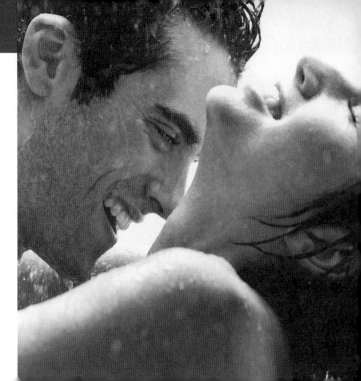

WATER+6+9

How does this sound? We shower, wash and dry one another. We get into bed, kiss, stroke, and nibble. Then, I'll spin around so that we can enjoy some slow, lingering, mutual oral sex. We're not going for orgasms, we're just going for pleasure. Maybe, pull me on top, but still no rush.

Then I'll lie next to you and we can breathe, before we move on... or sleep.

A REAL RIP OFF

We've all seen those movies where the couple is so passionate they rip the clothes off one another, which is fine when the wardrobe department is providing the clothes. In real life, you might not want to sacrifice that new outfit to the moment. Even so, the idea seems fun. So, how about a little advance planning for that evening when you want your man to tear your clothes off?

We all have clothes we won't miss. Of course, some things don't tear that easily, even T-shirts. So, you might even take a pair of scissors, and cut some tiny slits in the neckbands and waistbands to facilitate the ripping.

Anyway, it's all for fun. You'll either end up laughing, or feeling very passionate. Both are good.

Tear my clothes off…

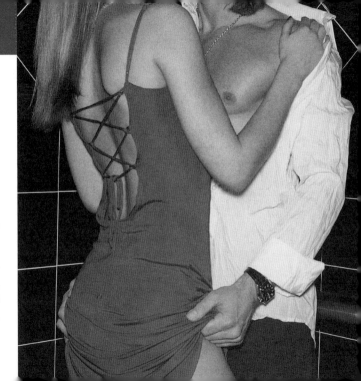

A REAL RIP OFF

Remember those good old B-movies where he wants her so much that he tears her clothes off? Well, we can be just as passionate as those actors.

If you notice tonight that I'm wearing an older outfit, it's because it's an outfit that no one will miss if it happens to get ripped in an evening of passion. Go on...tear my clothes off...I want you to.

EVERY NIGHT

So, what is the national average for a couple like you? Once a week, twice a week? We all seem to want to compare ourselves with others. Well, forget about that. Here is a little experiment that is meant to increase the quality of your intimacy through volume.

The idea is to agree with your partner that you will have sex every night for one week. It's not a marathon, and crossing the finish line each night is not the point. The point is to be physically intimate every night so as to recondition your thinking of sex as intercourse and orgasms.

Again, intimacy is the point. You might have full sex, just oral sex, just kissing and touching, mutual masturbation, massage, or being naked and just holding one another. It's not the outcome that is important. It's the communion.

Let's be intimate every night...

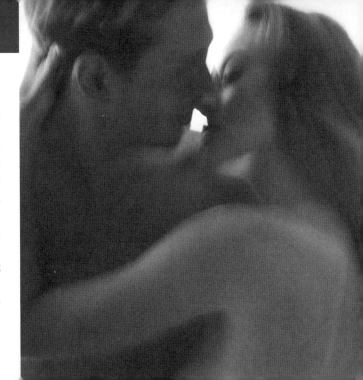

EVERY NIGHT

I have an adventure for us. It involves making love every night for one week. We will start tonight, and for seven days we will be intimate every night. We can have full sex, or get naked and just hold each other. We can massage each other, have oral sex, or whatever suits us. Most nights, we won't finish, just stop and sleep. One week of sexual, sensual, physical communion.

TIED UP

As much as you enjoy the mutual aspects of your sex life with your partner, the idea of being held captive and powerless, of being the complete focus of your lover's attention can be a powerfully erotic situation.

You will need something soft, like old neckties or scarves, or even torn up T-shirts. Have those available when the two of you get into the bedroom. The idea is that he ties your wrists and ankles to the corners of the bed or headboard. If your bed doesn't allow for that, he could tie your arms over your head or behind your back. You can only lie there, powerless, the center of his attention, as he takes you.

You captivate me....

TIED UP

Being held captive is an intriguing and erotic fantasy. If you happen to see some old silk ties or scarves laid out in the bedroom, feel free to tie my hands and feet to the bed, or just tie my hands over my head. Capture me, and have your way with me.

The only condition is that if I am uncomfortable and I ask you to untie me, you will do so. But I expect it will be very fun.

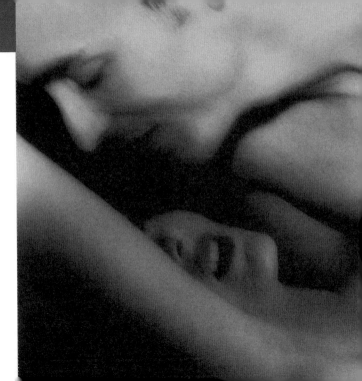

AFTERNOON DELIGHT

So many couples get in the habit, for obvious reasons, of making love as the last thing of the day. When they finally get in bed, as the day is done, they finally focus on each other. Even if you are not in that pattern, it's likely that you make love at a similar time of day each time. Just for a change, have a day when you shake up the clock. You might sneak in a date during your lunch hour, or before dinner, or before you go to work, or on a Saturday afternoon instead of Saturday night.

Making love when the sun is out may feel like something you're not supposed to be doing, but that's sort of the point. A few minutes of escape from your work and your daily routine will be making for a very memorable afternoon.

Pleasure while the sun shines...

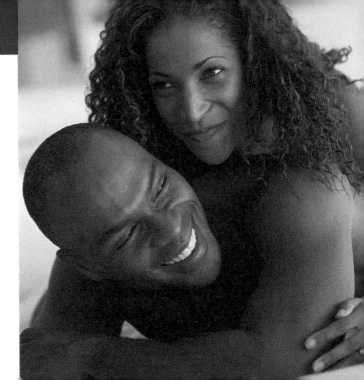

AFTERNOON DELIGHT

While the rest of the world is working and getting things done, let's sneak away, close the blinds, and get into bed for a daytime treat. We'll lock the door, not answer the phone for a few minutes, and wear a smile the rest of the day.

Tell me what's best for you, lunchtime, before dinner, or on a day off. Hmmm...sex while the sun shines.

I DON'T KNOW HOW

The two of you are familiar lovers; you know how to please one another. It wasn't always that way. In the beginning of your relationship, neither of you was completely sure of the best ways to please your partner.

Tonight, pretend it's the very beginning, at least for you. Meet him in bed with the idea that you know nothing about making love, nothing about his body or your own. Not that you'll be passive physically—you'll just let him guide you. Besides the fun you'll have playing innocent, you might learn ways to please him that you never knew about. This will not only be a fun game for you both, but might also make you better lovers.

Teach me how to please you....

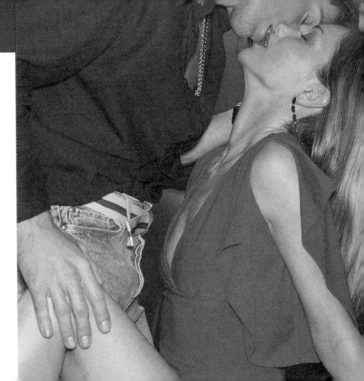

I DON'T KNOW HOW

I have a problem—I seem to have forgotten how to make love.

You're going to have to teach me everything. I'm a very good learner, so talk me through everything: if we should take things off, how we touch and what we touch, where and how I use my mouth...and all the other parts of my body.

LAST MINUTE SEX NOTE #1

When you have to have him, and you have to have him in a hurry, hand your man this sex note. You're in the mood, you aren't looking for a lot of ceremony or even a lot of romance. A quickie on the spot would be just the thing.

Enjoy.

Quick, I need you now...

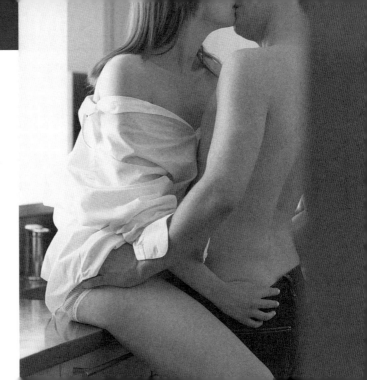

LAST MINUTE SEX NOTE #1

As soon as you finish reading this, we'll have a little race...to see who can get their clothes off the fastest.

We only have a few minutes, let's have some fast sex—a "quickie," I believe it's called. I'm ready now. Let's go.

LAST MINUTE SEX NOTE #2

Save this sex note as a surprise for when you are out together one evening, whether it's out to dinner, at a party, a movie, or anywhere with lots of people and fun. It should be a night when you are wearing a skirt or a dress. It will be a surprise to him, and a total turn on. People around you may wonder why you are smiling...and why you are leaving early.

I'll tell you my secret...

LAST MINUTE SEX NOTE #2

Sweetheart, how nice it is to be out with you. I thought you might enjoy knowing...I'm not wearing any underwear. Nothing.

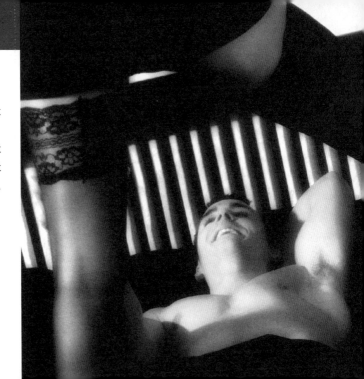

LOVE HER HAIR

Everyone loves attention; yet we are often self-conscious about asking for it. One of the simplest ways that you can give attention to the lady in your life is to pay attention to her hair. It may seem a simple thing to you, but she will love it if you offer to brush her hair. A little bit of pampering feels really good.

For a woman, so much of what is sexy is not actual sex but the ceremonies between men and women, before and after sex. This is a great ceremony, one that she will love. As simple as it seems, she will find it most romantic.

Let me play with your hair . . .

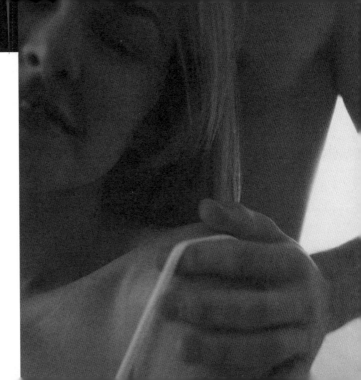

LOVE HER HAIR

This evening, whenever you are ready, I want you to bring your favorite hairbrush to me. Then I want to brush your hair for ten minutes or so. I'm not an expert, so feel free to guide me if I need help. I hope you'll find it relaxing. Afterward we can sleep or make love, whatever you feel like doing.

CUDDLE ME FIRST

Couples that have the good fortune of being together for awhile sometimes lose touch with the simpler physical moments of their beginning. After awhile, you tend to just start in the middle of lovemaking, skipping the preludes.

Although the talk shows make jokes about men not being good at cuddling, both of you will benefit from a return to some of your earliest forms of lovemaking. Frequently, the best way to heat up your sex life is to slow it down, and a few minutes of cuddling before you heat things up is a great way to do that. Make the house quiet, hold each other and talk, or just sit quietly and stroke one another. Recapture a simpler time in your relationship when this kind of physical communication was important.

Let's just cuddle...

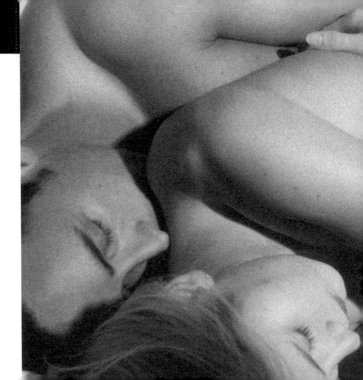

CUDDLE ME FIRST

Sweetheart, let's go back in time, to a moment when just holding one another was charged with electricity.

I certainly want to make love with you tonight, but let's first spend fifteen minutes of quality time just holding one another. We'll leave the day behind. Fifteen minutes of quiet, fifteen minutes of each other. A gentle and slow beginning to whatever follows.

UNDRESS FOR SUCCESS

Now that you've been together for awhile as a couple, when you go to bed together, you probably just get ready for bed separately and then meet in bed. Wouldn't it be nice to recreate some of the earlier anticipation and ceremony? What better way than to completely undress one another, deliberately, slowly, enjoyably.

If you have gotten into very casual clothes once you got home, when it's time, get dressed again. Put on some nice music, maybe some candles, and go through a ceremony undressing one another before you make love. Appreciate every bit of skin that is uncovered.

You'll have the double pleasure of spending the day thinking about it, and then doing it.

You undress me, I'll undress you...

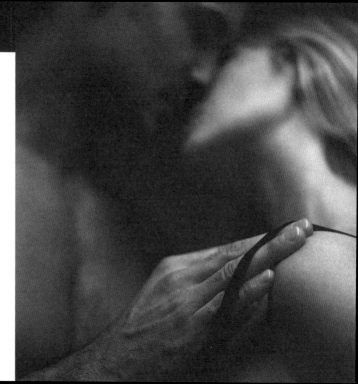

UNDRESS FOR SUCCESS

My darling, one of the ceremonies that we neglect these days is that bit of anticipation when the clothes are coming off. I want us to undress each other completely, before we make love. We'll put on some nice music, light a candle or two, and proceed to take everything off one another. It will be slow and deliberate, taking pleasure in the skin that is exposed with each item, never rushing.

INTIMACY Q & A

The intimacy that exists between a man and a woman when they are in bed together presents an opportunity for the exchange of ideas and intimate feelings that rarely exists in the day-to-day goings on. It's quiet; it's private; it's intimate.

The next time you are in bed together, put the books, TV, or usual rituals aside and use this rare opportunity to learn about each other with a few moments of question and answer. A few questions are suggested below, or you can provide your own. The point is to talk about things other than the business of the day. Spend a few minutes getting to know each other's minds, before you get on to knowing each other's bodies.

The sharing of your thoughts will improve the sharing of your bodies.

Intimacy is so much more than sex...

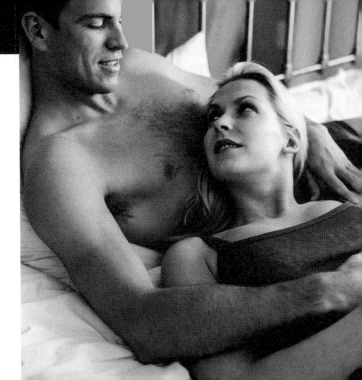

INTIMACY Q&A

I look forward to our time in bed. Tonight, let's share some thoughts we haven't shared before. We'll start with:

- Besides me, who was one of your greatest teachers in life?
- Is there a person whom you especially miss seeing?
- If you won a free trip to anywhere in the world, where would you want to go?

We'll have fun talking about these and then we can curl up together, make love, sleep, or whatever you would like.

HER ORGASM ONLY

Men are sometimes painted as being selfish in bed, but it's not really true. Most men very much want to satisfy their partner. Beyond the joy of knowing that she is happy, it's an incredible turn-on for a man to give his partner an orgasm.

Of course, both partners want their mate to have a "happy ending," but that desire can also be distracting. So, the next time you make love, dedicate the evening entirely to her pleasure, her orgasm. Let her know that you want her to be totally self-centered. We'll turn it around for you on another evening, but let her know that tonight is just for her. And let her have the option of sleeping afterwards, if that is what she wants to do.

Your selflessness will have many rewards.

It's all about your pleasure tonight...

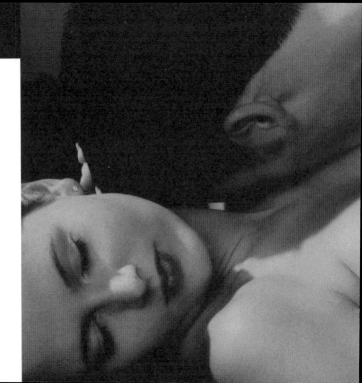

HER ORGASM ONLY

Darling, I know that you like to make me happy. Tonight though, I want to focus entirely on your pleasure, on your orgasm. I don't want you to think about my pleasure at all. As you feel your pleasure building, concentrate only on those sensations. Enjoy one orgasm, or several, or none. Whatever your body guides you to do, have some selfish pleasure.

PLEASURE HER FEET

Your feet are loaded with nerve endings, which many believe provide direct pathways to almost every part of your body. Massaging the feet potentially benefits your body in many ways—and at the very least, it feels wonderful. Massaging her feet is simple, requires almost no skill, and yet provides one of the most relaxing ways for her to end her day and begin a very sensuous evening.

Unless she's just out of the bath, put a towel under her feet and start with a wet, warm wash cloth. Gently clean and warm her feet. Then spread a small amount of oil or lotion on your hands, and just rub each foot. Technique is not overly important. Use long strokes or little circles, gently stretch her toes, and don't forget her heels. If she is ticklish, just slow down until she adjusts to your touch. Use the towel to dry and soothe her feet, and then move up to join her relaxed and invigorated body.

Let me rub your sweet feet...

PLEASURE HER FEET

My dear, when the day is done, how about I take those hardworking feet of yours and give you a foot massage. I will bring a towel and some lotion, and give your feet some much-deserved attention. Feel free to doze off, if you like. Of course, if you are still awake when I finish with your feet, we can think of some other way to give you pleasure.

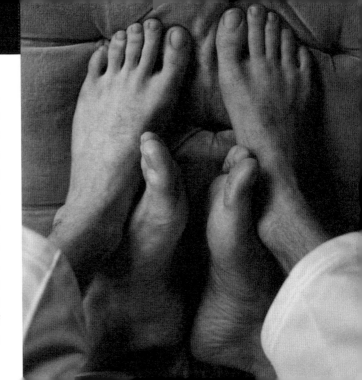

HOW ABOUT THE BACK SEAT?

In your earliest days of dating and sexual exploration, the car was an exciting, if not very comfortable, semi-private place for romance. Now that you live together and have a bedroom, the car is probably the last location you would pick for sex. But for a bit of fun—and yes, romance—get in your car for some parking.

It's a shame that drive-in movies are gone, but it will probably be better to just leave the car in the garage, or in the driveway. Anywhere that you have privacy and won't be interrupted. Take her by the hand, make your way into the car, and have some totally fun sex. It won't be any more comfortable than it ever was, but it'll be great fun nevertheless.

Let's go parking…

HOW ABOUT THE BACK SEAT?

Come with me into the past. Let's go "parking." I know that you never had a boy try to kiss you in the car, and I certainly never did anything like that, but I've heard that people have had a lot of fun in cars. So later, I'm going to take you by the hand, and we'll sneak into the back seat of the car for a little fooling around.

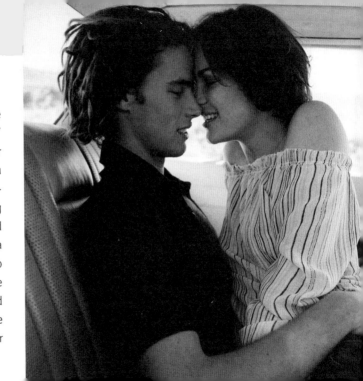

SCRITCH, SCRATCH

Women are good at so many things. Of course, they have specialized equipment that helps them sometimes—like those fingernails. When they apply them lightly to your skin, they can really give you chills, the good kind. You can do that for her as well, even if your nails aren't just right for the job. You'll have the fun of exploring her body, and she'll get all of those sensory awakening tingles.

If your nails aren't properly groomed for the job, locate a couple of tools, like a really soft hairbrush—maybe one with the rubber bristles—or you could use a loofah bath sponge. When the two of you are in bed, start with her back, and then cover her entire body with very light scratching, alternating with soft silky strokes. She'll be relaxed, yet tingling, with senses wide awake.

Let me make your skin tingle...

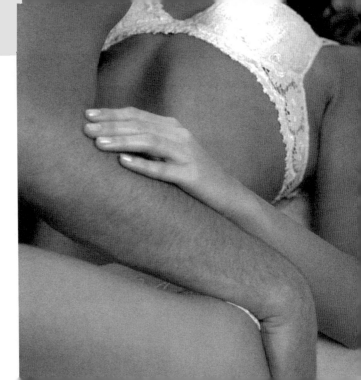

SCRITCH, SCRATCH

Sweetheart, when you scratch my back, it feels so very good. Tonight, I plan to gently scratch your entire body when we get into bed. I don't have your nails, so, I'll improvise, gliding gently across your bare skin in slow circles and long strokes, lightly scratching your neck, scalp, back, and everything down to your toes—first down your back side and then up your front.

PICK A POSITION

Every couple tries to keep some variety going. Even so, we all have positions for sex that seem to work best, or that we are just more used to, depending on our mood and energy level that night. We even have the side of the bed that we usually start from.

When you get into bed together tonight, start everything off differently than you usually would. Get on different sides of the bed, to begin with, and then talk to one another about one position for sex that is most always your favorite. Then talk about an alternate position that you think is funny, or particularly exciting, or one that you've never tried but want to. When the evening is over, you will hopefully know more about each other, and will have had some excitement or maybe some laughs.

New positions...

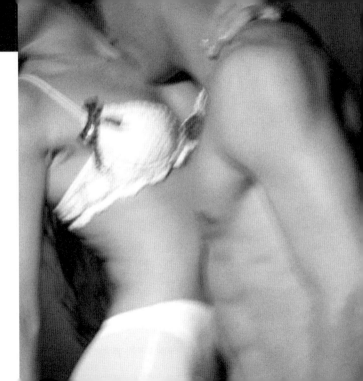

PICK A POSITION

The next time we make love, let's vary things, just for the fun of it. First, we'll start in different places on the bed, different sides, what ever is a change.

Then, we'll pick two sexual positions each, and talk about them. First, which position is our favorite, and why. Then, a position we've rarely or never tried. Then we'll play.

LOOK, NO HANDS

Lovemaking is always wonderful, but there's added fun when it's different. This note should be fun and interesting, as well as a challenge.

The next time you make love, don't use your hands, at least not to touch one another. The possibilities are limited only by your imagination. Of course, you might have to use your hands to undress and position yourself, but otherwise, let every other part of your bodies do the work. Caress her face and her breasts with your face, her back with your chest. Use your hair, your feet, your arms, your penis and, of course, your mouth.

Just don't use your hands.

Anything but hands on you tonight...

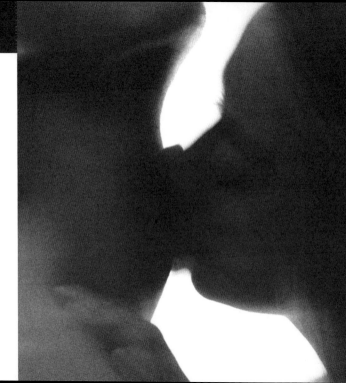

LOOK, NO HANDS

Darling, I love your hands on me, and mine on you. But there are so many other possibilities for using the rest of our bodies. Let's make love without using our hands. I'll stroke your face and breasts with my face, your back with my chest. I'll tickle your stomach and the insides of your legs with my hair. My lips, teeth, and tongue will take the place of my hands on every part of you.

SHE LIKES IT SLOW?

Women like things slow and easy; they like it soft and romantic—or so the story goes. However, it may be there are times when the woman you know wants it right now, and not so smooth. Perhaps there are times when she would rather you weren't the gentleman you are, and instead you just bent her over something and took her right then and there.

Moods do change, so this sex note is for her to hang onto until that time when slow and easy isn't what she's in the mood for. She may never use it, or then again, she might want more copies of it.

When you want to do me…now…hard and fast…

SHE LIKES IT SLOW?

My dear, I know that women are soft and romantic and that they want to be cared for, caressed, and gently loved. But I think there are also times when a woman doesn't want all of that nice womanly stuff. There are times when you just want it.

So, when you find yourself thinking "do me...now...hard and fast," just hand me this note. Whenever you want it.

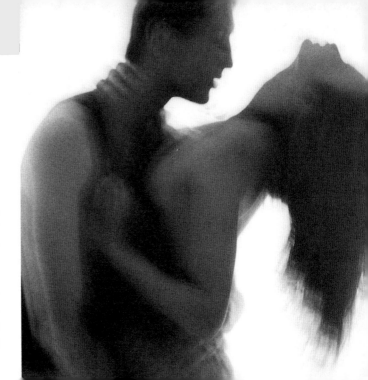

BATHING

You have undoubtedly noticed that she makes more of a ceremony out of bathing than you do. Men mostly take showers to get clean. Women get more than that out of their baths. It's a place to unwind, a place of serenity. It's also quite sensuous.

Tonight, invite yourself into her world of relaxation; join her in her bath. Make sure that there is some bubble bath, a washcloth or two, and to set a nice mood, find a couple of candles to light the room. It's a great place to get quiet together, and at the same time, to pamper her. Don't make it about a sexual experience, but rather a sensuous experience.

Let me pamper you . . .

BATHING

My dear, I can't help but notice how you enjoy your bath time. So, I would like to join you in your ceremony. It may be a little crowded, but I'll sit behind you and be your pillow.

When you are ready for your bath, I'll get the water going, and maybe find a candle or two. Then we can sit together and unwind.

See you in the tub.

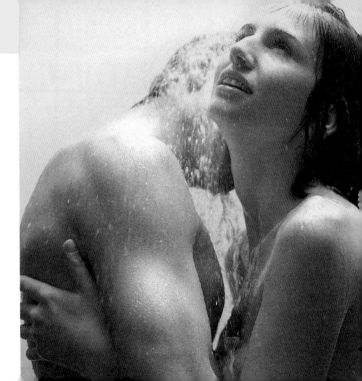

SLOW IT DOWN

One of the patterns that we fall into with our lovemaking is to move to that very enjoyable end result too quickly. In our lives, we're always being told to slow down and smell the roses. And so it should be with sex.

So, the next time you and your partner make love, let her know that you plan to break things up. After the two of you are nicely started, take a break, sit back, and slowly massage some part of her—her back, her chest, her arms. Take extra time kissing those same parts as you stroke them with your hands. It will give you a chance to touch and to view that body that you enjoy so much, and it will give each of you more time to build your pleasure and enjoy the moment.

Let me take my time with you...

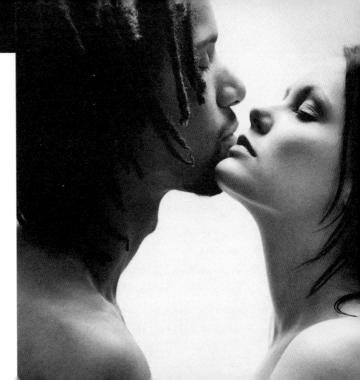

SLOW IT DOWN

Sometimes I don't take enough time when we make love. So, at some point in the middle of our lovemaking, I'm going to stop for a few moments. I'm going to sit back, enjoy the sight of you, then use my hands to massage some part of your wonderful body.

Then, when we do want to move on, we'll do so with a heightened sense of pleasure and awareness.

PLEASURE HER HANDS

Most women know the pleasure of a hand massage, because it's a part of getting her nails done at that nail salon. The better the salon, the better the hand massage, which is part of the reason they are willing to pay to go there. Having someone massage your hands is blissful, and not something we can do for ourselves. Receiving that massage from the person who cares most about you is even better.

So, if you want to give her a treat that she will remember, give her a hand massage. It takes no special talent, technique isn't overly important. Using whatever lotion you have, stretch and gently bend her hands, rub each finger, and massage almost up to her elbows.

You will make her feel cared for, relaxed, and happy. What better way to start a night together?

Let me massage your lovely hands...

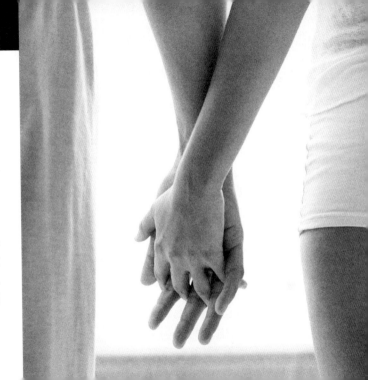

PLEASURE HER HANDS

I want to do something for a part of you that does so much, especially for me, a part that doesn't get enough attention—your hands. I am going to take your hands in mine and do my best to soothe the day away. I want you to lie back, close your eyes, and enjoy the sensations.

TOUCHING HER OTHER PLACES

Every couple gets to know their partner's body, and the best places to touch to give pleasure. Over time, you both tend to forget about the areas of your bodies that aren't the hot spots. Early in your relationship, you may have given great attention to her neck, arms, ears, the backs of her knees, and all of those other delicious places. You used to spend more time working up to the main event, building excitement, creating desire.

Here's a way to go back in time to those earlier lusty sessions. The next time you make love, kiss and stroke everywhere on her body, but don't touch the hot spots at all, at least not for a good while. Find them again, so that when you do finally get to her nipples, her vagina, and her clitoris, you will both already be turned on and very ready.

Let me explore your whole body....

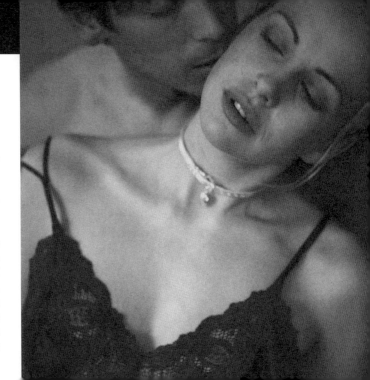

TOUCHING HER OTHER PLACES

My dear, remember the early days, when our hands and mouths explored our bodies, careful not to get to the most intimate spots too early. Anticipation was the key, nothing was routine, no conclusion automatic.

The next time we make love, I'm going to try to create that again. I may get close, but I am not going to touch the most intimate spots until much later, until you tell me you have to have me...there...now.

SEPARATE, THEN COME TOGETHER

Variety is the spice of life. Yes, but with sex we often fall into patterns of familiarity that feel comfortable and sure. Shake up your routine.

The next time you make love, when you are both quite excited, pull away from one another, and use your own hands to continue the pleasure, each watching the other please their own body, until you climax together, yet apart. By getting fully turned on together first, you will limit the inhibitions you might feel about masturbating in front of one another. And the visual excitement of witnessing one another's pleasure while so close together will create a very memorable night. Masturbation is usually solitary and private, and the openness of sharing it will not only be very exciting, but can bring you closer together as well.

Let me watch you take your pleasure...

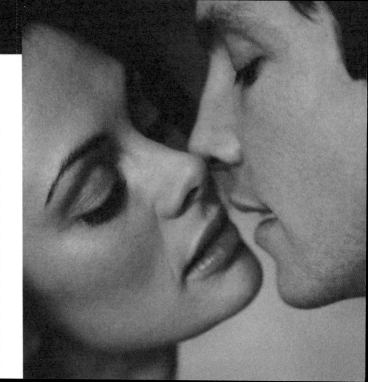

SEPARATE, THEN COME TOGETHER

Tonight, I want us to share what would usually be a private enjoyment. I want to begin together, kissing and touching and bringing each other to breathless excitement. Then, I would like to lean back and watch each other as we continue the pleasure with our own hands, slow and steady, with matching intensity. The excitement of sharing such a private moment will leave us breathless and add to the intimacy we already share.

BODY CONSCIOUSNESS

You often see her naked, and of course she sees you. Even now, there may be some self-consciousness, because you know that neither of you is perfect. She may feel she is in a competition with those images of models in every magazine and TV show, and may not know how much she excites you. And of course, you don't mind hearing that you do it for her as well.

So tonight, take the time to see, and to appreciate one another. With some gentle lighting in the room, explore. Find the parts you are not so familiar with. The back of the neck, the sole of a foot, between your fingers, the curve of the waist.

Tell each about favorite places on each of your bodies. The point is to notice and be noticed, but mostly, to appreciate.

Let's get naked and just explore...

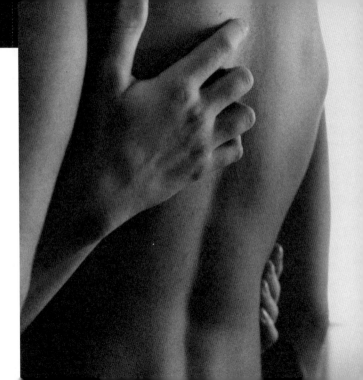

BODY CONSCIOUSNESS

We often see each other naked, and yes, we're flawed and imperfect. Tonight, before bed, let's explore that nakedness. We'll just roam around one another's bodies with our eyes and fingers. You tell me your two favorite places on your own body and on mine, and I'll do the same. We may not have bodies like models in magazines, but it's not those bodies that turn me on—it's yours.

A SPECIAL MASSAGE FOR HER

Everybody loves to be massaged. Isolating one area is more manageable than a full-body massage and requires no special training. This one should relax her and stimulate both of you.

Concentrate your full attention on the front of her body between her navel and her knees. It should be sensuous first and sexual second. Long, slow, and fairly deep strokes with lubricated hands along the sides of her hips and thighs, and back up slowly between her legs. Work gradually closer to the whole pubic area, and when you get there, start by using a flattened palm to gently press and massage the whole area. You will get to her vagina, but keep the strokes slow and steady, stroking the lips, massaging her clitoris.

Your intention should be a sensual massage more than sexual stimulation. The stimulation will happen anyway, and will be increased by her state of relaxation.

Erotic massage just for you…

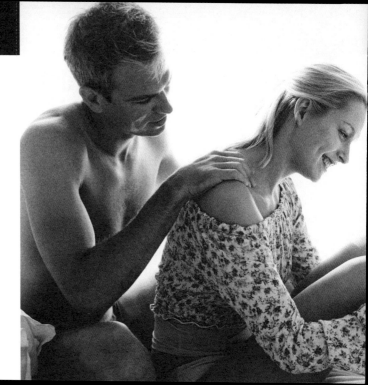

A SPECIAL MASSAGE FOR HER

I want to give you a sensuous and relaxing massage from your navel to your knees. I'll slowly stroke your thigh muscles and the sides of your hips and the insides of your legs. Eventually, I'll move my attention to that beautiful triangle between your legs, massaging the whole area.

My intention will not be to stimulate you sexually, but rather to relax you and arouse you into a sensual state.

CONTROL #1

For many men, the workday is comprised of schedules, deadlines, and having to meet expectations. When they get home, it could be nice to have a reprieve from the pressure and expectation of the workday, especially when they get to the bedroom. Whether this is your situation or not, giving over complete control to your partner for everything that happens in the bedroom can provide for a very pleasurable night.

For one evening, allow her to set the stage and control the entire outcome of your sexual meeting. Allow yourself to be completely passive in terms of directing the moment together, while being fully active in taking part in the enjoyment. Take a vacation from personal expectations.

You take control tonight...

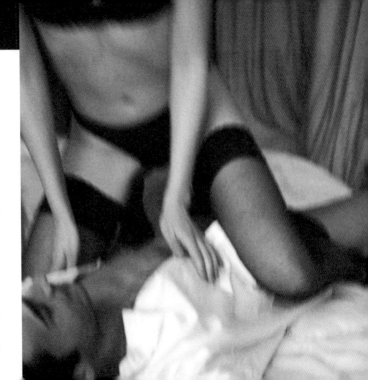

CONTROL #1

I know that you are aware of the tension I sometimes feel at work, making decisions, meeting other people's expectations, meeting deadlines. So, if you will indulge me, I would love to take one night off from being the man.

The next time we make love, I want to give myself over completely to you. Tell me what you want, where you want me. I will follow your lead, accept your desires and commands.

CONTROL #2

On the other hand, there may be days when your sex drive is strong and you want to lead the two of you in mutual pleasure, to take complete charge of the evening, sensually and sexually. If you think this would please her as well, then this sex note is the one to give her.

Even though you want the pleasure to be mutual, let her know that you plan to guide the experience, to set the stage. Take charge of the whole experience. You can run a bubble bath for her, and be waiting with a robe. Guide her to the space you have planned, and have the candles lit. Dress her as you wish, or not. Have some oil ready, if you wish, and maybe a glass of wine. Whatever you imagine as an enjoyable sexual and sensual evening for her to enjoy.

Tonight, I'm in control...

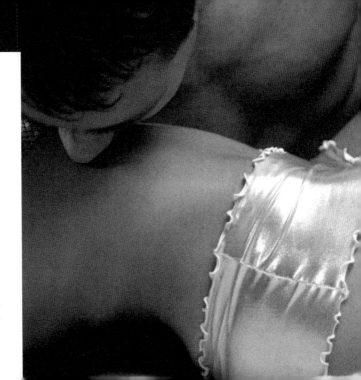

CONTROL #2

My darling, I know your day is nonstop, working and planning, taking care of yourself and me and everything else you do, all the while being my sensuous, loving partner.

For tonight, I want you to put no effort into that last part, except to enjoy yourself. I'm going to take control of the evening in that area. I'll take the lead, you only need to take pleasure.

DON'T FINISH TONIGHT

For a man, there is a certain amount of focus on the orgasm itself. It is the desired and expected goal of sex together. To have sex and not have an orgasm might be slightly foreign and, perhaps, frustrating. But it could also be liberating to make love without your orgasm as a goal. It will certainly provide a dynamic and differently paced experience of lovemaking if you start with the idea that you aren't going to come.

You'll end the evening in a very heightened state of sensuality, anticipating your next meeting together. Believe me, it's an experience worth having.

I'm saving my pleasure for later...

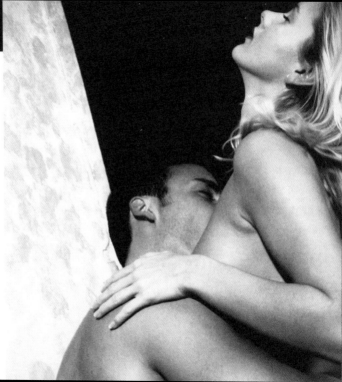

DON'T FINISH TONIGHT

For one evening, I want to make love with you without having an orgasm. But, you should come as early and as often as you wish. I think it will make for a differently paced and very playful evening.

To keep from coming, I might have to stop and start over again a few times. That could make for an extended evening of pleasure for you. I hope you don't mind.

A TASTE OF HER

Oral sex. It's great. To receive, to give...it's all good.

With all sex, of course, we try to give mutual pleasure, to satisfy one another, to take turns in the enjoyment. But it's also nice to have the gift of just receiving. So, make this a night just for her to receive. After all, you get the pleasure of her pleasure.

I want to taste you...

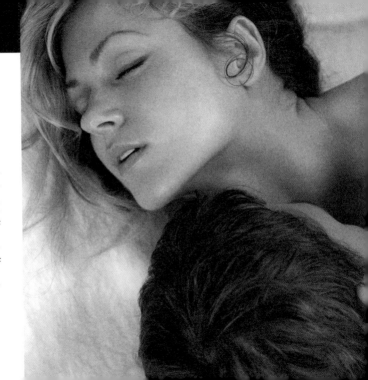

A TASTE OF HER

Tonight, let's make it your turn, with no need to be mutual or to trade off. I'll be happy to take my turn or join in mutual oral pleasure another time, but for tonight, I just want the pleasure of my lips on your skin, exploring every inch of your wonderful body, tasting its sweetness.

IN PUBLIC

If you have been together as a couple for awhile, you probably don't have the public displays of affection you once did. But new couple or old, there is still a thrill in getting away with something that you usually reserve for more private moments.

The next time you plan a night out, let your lady know that you will be looking for moments to touch. You will be discreet, of course, stealing a touch in the elevator as others stand nearby, or riding in the cab, sitting in traffic, on a crowded street, or a deserted corner. It will be a shared game, which will leave you laughing and turned on and feeling younger in your relationship.

It will be an adventurous shared secret, and very sexy.

I can't keep my hands off you....

IN PUBLIC

I'm looking forward to going out with you tonight. And I want to go back in time, when neither of us could keep our hands away, even in public.

I won't embarrass us, or get us arrested, but I will be looking for moments to touch you and play with you. Wear something that allows me to find your skin more easily please. It will be an adventure, a secret between us.

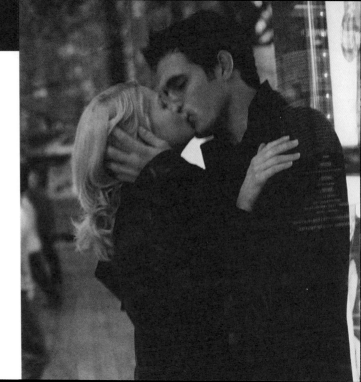

TELL ME WHAT YOU WANT

No matter how great a relationship you have, or how great the sex is, there will be certain desires, spontaneous thoughts, or temporary moods that one isn't sure how to express to their partner, especially when it comes to lovemaking. It may be even harder for a well established couple to say something, for fear of sounding critical or that the other might think they have been doing it wrong all along.

If you make it clear that you want to know, and if you keep comments positive, the relationship will benefit.

Let her know that you really want to hear her inner thoughts, secret wishes, and sudden desires. She may find it difficult to be overly verbal, but your willingness to listen will be a welcome show of affection. Your relationship will benefit, and it may provide for a very sexy evening.

Your wish is my command...

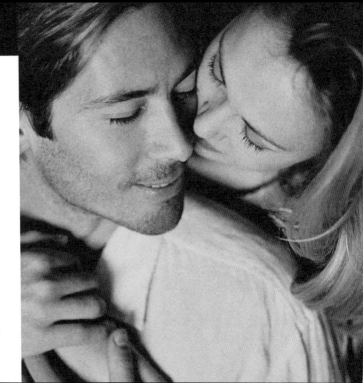

TELL ME WHAT YOU WANT

Next time we are making love, I want you to tell me what you want. I would love to hear you say something like, "I like that, I want to feel what it's like when you do it faster/slower." Or maybe, "You know what we've never done before..." Or maybe just, "Would you...?"

I'll listen. I want to know what you like and what you want, even if you only want it tonight.

HAND JOB FOR TWO

When we start making love, we usually have a goal in mind, a picture of that excellent ending. Whatever happens before, intercourse is probably where we are headed. However, it can be both exciting and liberating to plan a different ending.

Making love and touching one another, we sometimes fail to linger as we might on a moment of pleasure. Our thoughts are on moving to the next step.

This time, as your hands focus on one another's genital pleasure, really focus on that. Allow yourselves to climax using your hands only. Enjoy the variety of ways you can give and take pleasure. Play together, take turns. Have some light oil nearby, if you like, to add to the pleasure. Take your time with it, and enjoy the ending.

I love my hands on you. I love your hands on me...

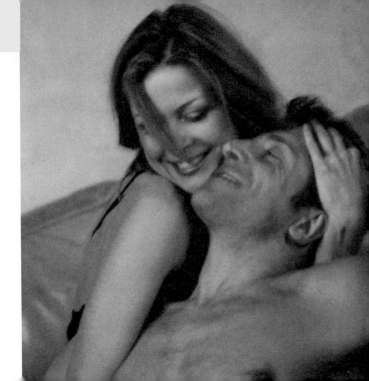

HAND JOB FOR TWO

I love my hands on you. I love your hands on me. Even so, we might not pay full attention to the pleasure our hands can give. So that we focus on this pleasure, I propose a no intercourse rule tonight. At a moment when we might join our bodies together, we'll concentrate on bringing one another to climax using our hands.

I can't wait to be in your hands.

KISSING

It is said that women, especially, like to kiss. If that's the case, go with it.

When you first met one another, you could have kissed for hours. You probably did. So, indulge her pleasure once again, and enjoy the rewards. Have an old fashioned make out session. Many of us just don't give enough attention to kissing and the pleasures it brings.

She will appreciate your attention, I guarantee.

Just kissing you is making love...

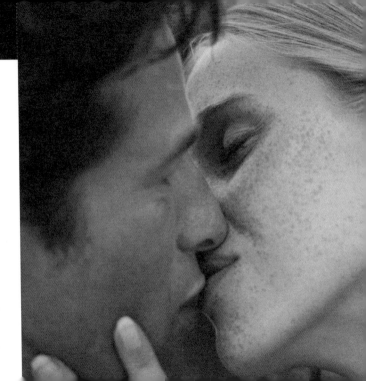

KISSING

Kiss me. Hmmm...that's nice. Remember when we first met? I could have kissed you for hours. I think I did.

Perhaps now we don't give enough attention to the pleasure of kissing one another. So, tonight, before we move into the bedroom, let's get a glass of something nice to drink, and spend some time sitting together and kissing. Really kissing. Let's make out.

A LIGHT TOUCH

We sometimes forget that simply changing the pressure of our touch and kisses can bring delightful new experiences. Letting your fingers and lips move slowly and with very light pressure can build excitement and anticipation.

The next time the two of you are in bed together, soften your touch. As passion builds, we feel like touching more and harder and faster. Concentrate on letting your fingers and lips roam her entire body, but with a light and smooth motion. Keep your touch light and soft until she insists you touch her harder.

Although you don't want to turn your foreplay into tickling, a light and deliberate touch will build anticipation, focus the sensations, and extend the pleasure of the evening. At some point, of course, the tempo will pick up, but allow yourself to linger, and enjoy.

I'm going to linger on you...

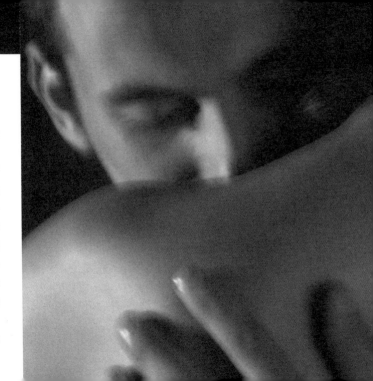

A LIGHT TOUCH

Tonight, my sweet one, I plan to touch you with the gentlest and lightest of touches. I am going to linger on every part of you with my fingers and my lips. In the excitement of making love with you, I sometimes fail to linger in the pleasure of touching you with a slow and gentle hand.

I hope you enjoy a lighter touch.

A BACK RUB, AND MORE

This is pure pleasure. After you are in bed together, and naked, invite her to lie on her stomach. Have some oil nearby, and sit straddling her legs. Apply a fair amount of oil to her back, your hands, your stomach, and your penis. Then, slowly begin to massage her back. Technique isn't important, just stroke her muscles, and up and down along her spine.

For the "more" part, let your body begin to get involved in the stroking, allowing your stomach and penis to join in the massage. Slowly, very slowly, let your penis begin to slip between her legs. Keep the massage going as you begin to slowly enter. Allow the progression to intercourse to take a long time, and continue rubbing her back the whole time, blending the two actions.

This is pure pleasure, for both of you.

Pure pleasure for us both...

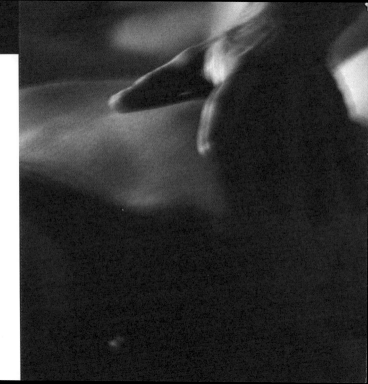

A BACK RUB, AND MORE

I have an idea for this evening, which I believe will be pure pleasure for us both. I want to give you a back rub...and more.

After I oil your back and my hands, I'll begin stroking your back. As you enjoy my hands and the relaxation they offer, slowly, ever so slowly, I will slide between your legs, and we'll blend massage and lovemaking...warm, sensuous, slippery, and slow.

MIRROR, MIRROR

There is little denying the power of visuals in sex. Just seeing her naked gets the motor running. The pleasure of seeing yourselves joined in lovemaking is an absolute turn on. Mirrors on ceilings are mostly in the movies, most people don't have a mirror that is trained on their bed, but you can improvise.

Somewhere in your home, you have a framed mirror that you can temporarily move to your bedside, or you might choose to take her to where the mirror is hanging.

Whatever you can arrange mirror wise, spend a few minutes setting a mood, maybe a candle or two, or some subtle lighting. Then, the two of you can just enjoy the view.

A truly beautiful sight...us, making love...

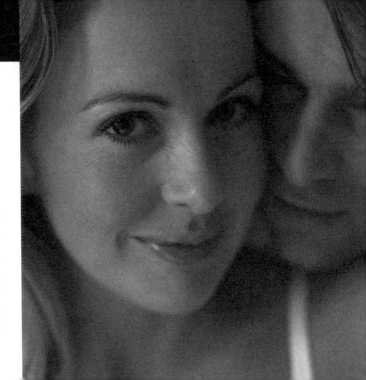

MIRROR, MIRROR

If I haven't told you lately, I love the sight of you. Your body is a feast for my eyes. Seeing us together is a thrill.

I want to set a mirror someplace by the bed, just for tonight, so that we can enjoy a truly beautiful sight...us, making love. We could also move our activities to a mirror somewhere in the house, if you prefer. I can't wait to see us.

AURAL SEX

You may be a terrific communicator, but some men aren't. Either way, we all take for granted that our partner "knows how I feel," especially if we have been together for awhile. As good as we might be at making love physically, most of us neglect making love with our words.

The next time you are together in bed, set the mood with some quiet music, and let her know the things that you appreciate about her, her body, your relationship. As you make love, stop and find places on her body that you love, the shape of her ears, the curve of her waist, the shape of her breasts. Tell her, "I love it when you..." Dedicate yourself to saying at least ten positive things about her, and about your feelings for her. You may think she knows these things; but she wants to hear them. You will be rewarded.

Let me whisper in your ear...

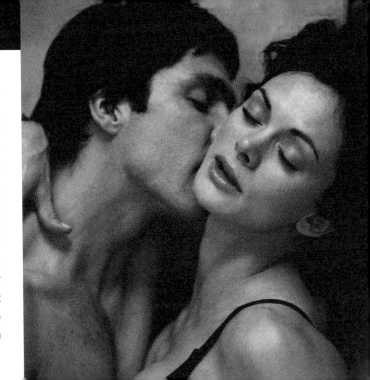

AURAL SEX

I probably don't always let you know how I feel. I assume you know, but you might like to hear the words. Things I love about us, about you, your mind and body, how good you make me feel. So, tonight, I'm going to tell you some of those things. I may be better with my hands, but tonight, I am going to make love to you with my words.

ORAL SEX

Oral sex, as part of foreplay leading to intercourse, is terrific. But it's also terrific to luxuriate in those oral sensations with no thought of moving on to anything else. So, the next time you make love, suggest to her that you do just that. It can be mutual, but let her know that as much as you enjoy her attention, you want to focus on her pleasure and to take your time with her. Use your mouth and tongue slowly and lightly, making sure not to rush anything. Let her body relax into your attentions. Your orgasm is more likely to bring an end to the evening than hers is, so allow yourself to hold off as long as possible in reaching your own peak.

She won't forget your attentions.

I love to kiss and nibble and taste every part of you....

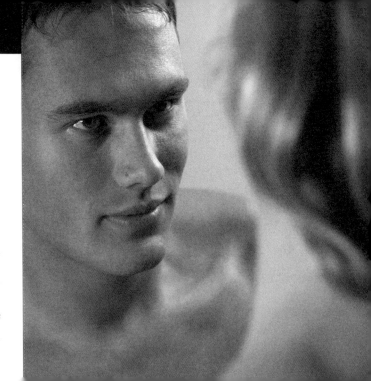

ORAL SEX

You give me so much pleasure when we make love, I feel selfish sometimes. I wonder if my mouth gives you nearly as much pleasure as yours gives me. Tonight, I want our lovemaking to be only oral sex. It can be mutual, but let me take my time with you first, and allow your body to completely relax into the sensations of my mouth on you. I can't wait.

I'M NEW AT THIS

At this point as a couple, you know quite well how to please one another. But think back to the beginning of your relationship, or even to when you were a complete novice sexually. At that point you were just excited and happy to be there, unaware of the best ways to please a partner.

Tonight, pretend it's the very beginning, at least for you. Meet her in bed with the idea that you know nothing about making love, nothing about her body or your own. Not that you'll be passive, you'll just let her guide you. Besides the fun you'll have as she teaches you to make love, you may learn ways to please her that you never knew about. Not only will this be a fun game for you both, but it will perhaps even make you better lovers.

Show me exactly how you want it...

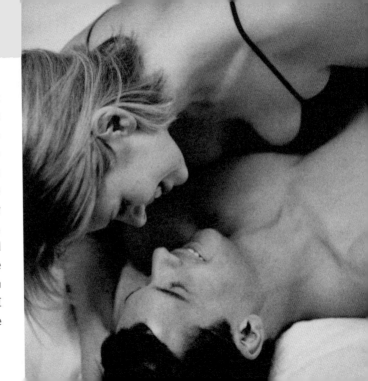

I'M NEW AT THIS

My dear one, I know that I want to make love with you, but I seem to have forgotten everything about how to do it. Please teach me to make love with you, how to kiss, where to touch, and how. I'm a good learner, so all you have to do is talk me through it and show me what I should do. Teach me everything.

WHAT'S YOUR PREFERENCE?

Everyone's mood changes from day to day, and communicating those moods is one of the challenges for a couple, especially when it comes to the bedroom. You have a list of preferences on all of the functions of your computer, which you can adjust anytime you wish. Just for fun, why not have a preference list for your partner to check off the next time you are in bed together. It's serious, it's honest, but mostly, it's just fun.

She can bring this list to bed, or convey it to you beforehand. Either way, you'll have a great time going through her preferences.

Tell me what you want....

WHAT'S YOUR PREFERENCE?

Please check, or mark in 1-2-3 order, your love-making preferences, for tonight only:

___Play with my breasts
___Kiss my neck
___Go down on me
___Play with my ass
___Cuddle with me
___Mutual oral sex
___Spank me a little
___I want it from behind
___Nibble my ears
___Rub my back
___I'll be on top
___other_____

A HAND FOR HER

We use our hands to bring wonderful pleasure to our partners, but it is usually a part of a progression toward intercourse. The experience of masturbation is perhaps more relaxed and simple, not a session of lovemaking, just the sensation of pleasure and relaxation.

Offer her that pleasure, only with you taking care of the handwork. Once you are together and have had a chance to relax, let her lean back against you as you sit in bed, and let your hands become hers, gently squeezing her breasts, stroking her belly and using your fingers to bring her pleasure. She should know that you don't mean for this to lead to anything. You just mean for it to be a gift of pleasure. She may come, or she may not. You just want her to relax and feel pleasure before you both go to sleep.

Tonight, let me offer you my hands...

A HAND FOR HER

Tonight, let me offer you my own hands to put you into a pleasure state before sleep. Once we are in bed, I'd love for you to just sit in front of me, lean back, and close your eyes. I'll wrap my arms around you and let my hands become yours, gently stroking and squeezing and pleasuring you. My only goal is for you to experience pleasure and relaxation before sleeping.

WE WON'T RUSH IT

Remember your early sexual days. Foreplay lasted forever. It was frustrating, but thrilling at the same time. For many couples, the longer you are together, the less time you dedicate to foreplay.

The goal here is to return some of the thrill and imagination of those earlier days, to break sexual routines and extend the whole experience of sex. This sex note will please her and hopefully recall some of the excitement and pleasure of an earlier time.

You will need a timing device, set for twenty minutes. Once you begin making love, don't allow intercourse to begin for the entire twenty minutes. It may seem like a long time compared to what you have become used to, but what a nice way to pass time. It will be worth the wait.

Let's take all the time in the world...

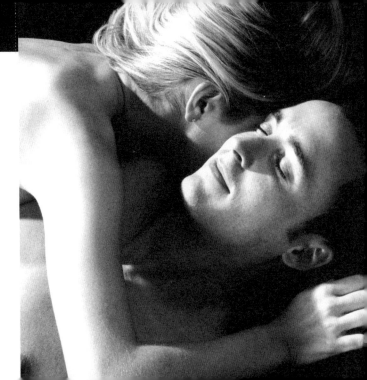

WE WON'T RUSH IT

I *love* the sex we have together, but I can recall earlier days together when we dedicated ourselves more to the thrill of foreplay. So, I propose we extend the time we spend working up to that big rush of pleasure.

I have a timer. Tonight, I propose we set it for twenty minutes, and once we begin making love, we will not allow any penetration until the timer runs out.

THE FULL BODY KISS

Kissing might be the most intimate expression of all.

Let her know that tonight you plan to kiss her. Kiss her from her toes to the top of her head. When the time comes, kiss her softly on the lips, and then guide her to lie face down, naked, on your bed. Begin with her toes and ankles, and kiss and nibble up to the backs of her knees. Maintain constant contact, at least with a hand. Continue up her legs and rear, striving for sensuous touch rather than sexual. Up to the back of her neck, and gently roll her over. Kiss her face softly, and move down her body. Refrain from oral sex, and continue to kiss down to her toes, slowly, gently, and deliberately...and enjoy the rest of the evening.

Let me kiss every part of you...

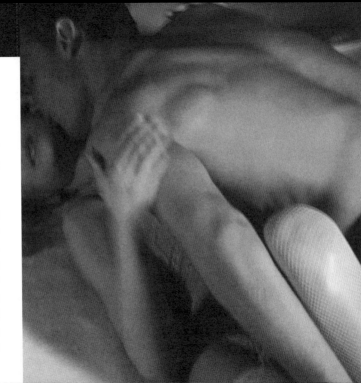

THE FULL BODY KISS

From now on, I want to avoid routines, and to touch more often. Above all, we should kiss every day. I'm talking about affectionate touching, and not necessarily sex. I'll go first, starting tonight, with a full body kiss. Your lips first, down to your toes, softly kissing my way up your back and neck to where I began. Then we'll sleep, or maybe make love. In my mind, I'm kissing you now.

LAST MINUTE
SEX NOTE #1

When you think about sex with your partner, you mostly think about things that feel good to you, that you like to do. For the most part, you know what she enjoys. But maybe she has a fantasy, or knows something that would surprise you. Most of us do have little things tucked away that we think about sometimes.

Let her fill in the blank; learn from her, about her. If what she says sounds wild to you, or if it sounds dull, don't raise your brow, have an opinion, or worry that somehow it reflects on you or your abilities. Maybe you are the rare couple that knows everything about one another, but it's unlikely. If she has it to teach, learn something new about her.

Enjoy the adventure.

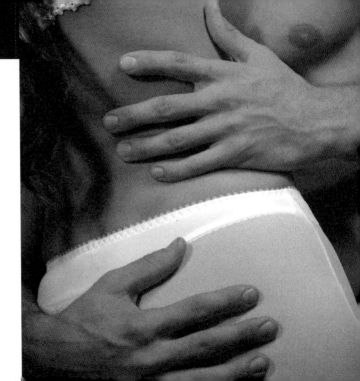

SPECIAL SEX NOTE #1

Tell me something that I don't know about you. Tell me something that I haven't thought of, or that you fantasize about, or that you read about or saw in a movie, or that you tried once and want to try again with me. You can use of the following leads:

• I've always wondered how it would feel to
  _____.

• I read this article about_____.
  I'd like to try that.

LAST MINUTE SEX NOTE #2

There are times when she is ready for some physical attention, but you are in the middle of something that perhaps she hesitates to interrupt. So, with her potential needs in mind, give her this note to use whenever she wants.

The deal is, whatever you are doing when she gives this sex note to you, you have to drop it for a little while. (If it's a game you have to see, start the VCR.) Look at it this way, you may miss a little of one thing, but in exchange, you get to have sex with the lady of your life, and you earn some major points.

Not bad!

I'll drop everything when you need me...

LAST MINUTE SEX NOTE #2

I know that there are times that you are ready for some physical attention, even though it's not our usual time, or it would interrupt something one of us is doing. No matter.

Save this note for whenever you want. I agree, in advance, to drop what I'm doing and join you for a little fun. The following words will remind me:

Darling, I need you for a few minutes.

Coming?

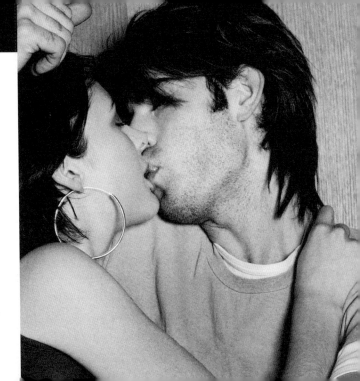

ABOUT THE AUTHOR

John Leslie Wolfe is an author, actor, and singer on Broadway and on television. He has performed in *Parade*, *Passion*, and *Evita*, and has also appeared in *The West Wing*, *Homicide*, and HBO's *Something the Lord Made*, in addition to a long list of commercial appearances.